# Intermittent Fasting Guide for Weight Loss

*The Ultimate Beginners Guide for Weight Loss, Heal Your Body, and Live a Healthy Lifestyle while Eating Your Favorite Foods (Includes 5:2 and 16:8 Method).*

**Dorothy Smith**

# Table of Contents

# Introduction

Thank you so much for purchasing the book. *Intermittent Fasting Guide for Weight Loss: The Ultimate Beginners Guide for Weight Loss, Heal Your Body and Live a Healthy Lifestyle while Eating Your Favorite Foods (Includes 5:2 and 16:8 Method).*

# Chapter 1: What Is Intermittent Fasting?

In this chapter, we will talk about intermittent fasting, and what it is, many people don't know, but intermittent fasting is one of the best ways to not only detoxify your body but to lose fat and build muscle. But there are many benefits to intermittent fasting, we will talk about all of those soon enough but let's just brief you on what is intermittent fasting. Intermittent fasting is a way for you to eat cyclically; it is mostly you starving yourself for 16 hours and then eating in an 8-hour window. Believe it or not, we used to do intermittent fasting back in the day. Our ancestors would be left without food for a couple of days, and once they would get the food, they would consume as much as possible so that they can store it and use that for energy.

As you know, they did not have access to grocery stores or restaurants where they could get food readily available, which is why they had to hunt for it, and when they did get the food, they would genuinely savor the food as much as possible. Evidently enough, our ancestors did not have diseases such as cancer or diabetes, and there's a reason for that. When we are fasting, our body is not producing that much insulin, which keeps our body insulin sensitive. It is essential to say insulin sensitive as it will help us tremendously with staying young while bettering our digestion of food once we do consume. Moreover, intermittent fasting helps you with reducing your cravings for sugar or anything unhealthy. Intermittent fasting is so good, many people who follow certain religions will fast for bettering themselves and self-control. Fasting has been a part of humans and human evolution, and there is a reason why many people who are very successful practice fasting as fasting has shown to help brain function and reduce mental fog. Time and time again, there has been scientific research showing how intermittent fasting can help you to not only better your brain function but to also help you with getting rid of brain fog.

As you know, brain fog has been an epidemic in our society, which is why getting rid of any brain fog can help us tremendously, which will not only our work but our performance outside of work. For example, let's say you're interested in farming, and you need to use hazardous tools to do so, the last thing you want is brain fog when operating these machines. Not only brain fog can reduce an individual's productivity, but it can be dangerous. Yes, that was an over-the-top example, but you can see how brain fog can have such a significant impact on our life. Intermittent fasting has also shown to reduce the risk of cancer, and there have been many scientific studies showing that intermittent fasting can boost your immune system and help you reduce the risk of cancer. There was one person who fasted for ten days non-stop, and he got rid of his cancer. Please don't quote me on this, but there have been some claims stating as such. However, there has been nothing but positive reviews with intermittent fasting. Now there are many ways for you to follow intermittent fasting. We will talk about in-depth later on in this book. However, the beautiful thing about intermittent fasting is that anybody can follow intermittent fasting does not matter what their lifestyle is and how they would like to go about following intermittent fasting. Intermittent fasting does not mess up your lifestyle; it, in fact, goes with your lifestyle depending on which type of protocol you follow. As long as you are following intermittent fasting for the right things, you will have no problem with achieving success, and now you might be asking why you should follow intermittent fasting and who it is for in terms of benefits. Let us break that down right now, to be fair, and this question is very vague, so we will try and answer the questions in different scenarios.

## Who Is Intermittent Fasting For?

Intermittent fasting is for people who are looking to lose fat and build muscle while optimizing your hormone and immune system. For example, let's say you are someone who's looking to better their health and live for a long time, the great thing about intermittent fasting is that it has been shown to increase your growth hormone production which will make you feel a lot younger. On top of that, intermittent fasting can also help you to boost your immune system, which will help you not only to lose fat but to build muscle. Also, if you're someone who's looking towards detoxifying themselves or their body, intermittent fasting can help you tremendously. Look at it like this, what better way to detoxify your body plan to cut out food source completely.

As you know, intermittent fasting helps you with the process of autophagy, which is a way for your body to get rid of any dead cells in your body. Intermittent fasting helps you with detoxing your body inside and out, which is why if you are someone looking to detoxify your body, then intermittent fasting is the way to go. If you are someone who's looking to increase their athletic performance, then intermittent fasting will be your savior. As you know, intermittent fasting has shown to increase your growth hormone levels and testosterone levels in men, which is why athletes need to practice intermittent fasting to a certain degree. Many professional basketball players and football players practice intermittent fasting, and they have seen amazing results. If you are someone looking to build up their discipline levels, then there is nothing better than intermittent fasting. The reason why intermittent fasting can be a great asset for people looking towards building discipline is that there is nothing more will power testing than someone who needs to eat food. If you're hungry. You can fight it off, then that will truly test your discipline level and will increase it if you follow intermittent fasting. Now that you know who should follow intermittent fasting, let's talk about the people who should not follow intermittent fasting.

## Who Should Not Follow Intermittent Fasting?

In specific scenarios, you should not follow intermittent fasting, so let's talk about people and circumstances where you should not follow intermittent fasting. If you're someone who's on diabetic medication, it is not advised for you to follow intermittent fasting. You see, when you're intermittent fasting, your body is not consuming any food for an extended amount of time. That is when your insulin level will altogether drop as your body has nothing to digest. If you're someone who has diabetes, you are not producing insulin; then, you need to be taking insulin regularly. If you take insulin while you're fasting, then you could go into a diabetic coma, which is something you don't want to mess with. Another scenario when people should not follow intermittent fasting is if your pregnant or are trying to get pregnant. This mostly applies to women; if you are someone who is trying to conceive or if you are pregnant, then intermittent fasting is not your savior. The reason why intermittent fasting is not suitable for you is that it can play a significant toll on your pregnancy and hormones. When you are pregnant, your hormones will be out of whack, so to speak, which is why it is imperative for you to eat regularly. It is also not advised for women too fast on a daily basis, but we will talk about that later on in this chapter in regard to how women should be intermittent fasting. The best advice we can give you is to consult with your doctor always when looking towards following intermittent fasting, as intermittent fasting can play a significant role in how you're going to be achieving your goals in regards to your fitness and health.

## Some Misconceptions

Now that you have a clear idea of what intermittent fasting is and who should follow it and who shouldn't let's talk about some of the misconceptions that you might hear about intermittent fasting. One of the many misconceptions about intermittent fasting is that women should not follow intermittent fasting. Now to a certain degree, that is true. If your pregnant are looking to conceive, then you should not follow intermittent fasting. However, women can follow intermittent fasting, but they need to be careful. This means that women cannot fast every day for the whole month; they should have certain days where they are consuming food regularly. This will ensure that there are hormones that don't go out of whack and that everything stays copacetic. There are many books on how women should follow intermittent fasting, and if you're a woman, then you will get a clear idea on how to follow intermittent fasting once you're done reading this book. However, if you still want to learn a little bit more, than we suggest you shop for a woman intermittent fasting books. Back to the topic, if you're a woman, then you should follow intermittent fasting but in a modified version.

Another thing women should understand is that if your pregnant or looking to conceive, then stay away from intermittent fasting as it can have havoc in your system. Another misconception with intermittent fasting is that you will lose muscle. The truth is intermittent fasting will help you to gain muscle when you're intermittent fasting, and your body is producing a lot more growth hormone 4000% more than you would normally. This increase in growth hormones can have a significant effect on how you put on muscle. Media has made you believe that you need to eat every two hours to maintain your muscle and to put on muscle. But the truth is that you can indeed put on muscle while following intermittent fasting as you will increase your growth hormone so much that you say anabolic the whole time. If someone tells you that intermittent fasting does not help you put on muscle, or it makes you lose your muscle mass. They don't know what they're talking about, as their much research has shown that intermittent fasting can increase your growth hormone and testosterone. And therefore help you to put on more

9

muscle and to preserve it. Another misconception you might have about intermittent fasting is that you can eat whatever you want during your eating window. The truth is that it is entirely false, if you're looking to lose weight, then you need to be in a caloric deficit while following intermittent fasting. It is simple math. If you think about it, the calories you burn need to be higher than then calories you consume. If you're following intermittent fasting to lose body fat, then we would highly recommend that you refrain yourself from consuming junk food and have healthy foods in a caloric deficit. These are mostly the misconceptions we hear about. With that being said, let's give our final verdict.

## Final Verdict

You should now know that intermittent fasting is something where you're eating cyclically, meaning that you will not eat for certain hours of the day and that you will eat in a particular eating window. Intermittent fasting can genuinely be a beneficial eating plan if you meet the criteria. If you're someone looking to put on more muscle, lose fat, or to increase your athletic performance, then intermittent fasting is your savior. Or if you're someone looking to detoxify your body, then there's nothing better to detoxify than intermittent fasting. If you're someone who's looking to decrease the risk of diseases that intermittent fasting is also the answer for you. There are many tremendous benefits which come along intermittent fasting, although it requires a lot more dedication it is still one of the best plants to follow when it comes to losing fat and building muscle while staying healthy. Please consult with your doctor before you follow intermittent fasting, even though it is such a great plan to follow it is not suited for certain people. As we told you, if your pregnant or looking to conceive, then intermittent fasting is not the answer for you, and if you're someone facing diabetes, then definitely consult with your doctor. With that being said, we now conclude this chapter.

# Chapter 2: Benefits of Intermittent Fasting

Now that you have a clear idea of what intermittent fasting is, let's talk about some of the benefits that come along with intermittent fasting. The truth is many benefits come along with intermittent fasting, and they have all of them backed up by science. Keeping that in mind, we will now talk about some of the significant benefits which come along with intermittent fasting so that you can get a better idea of why you should follow it and how it can be beneficial to you. One thing to remember is that all these benefits are great, but you must make sure that you are fit to follow intermittent fasting if you're not fit and healthy to support intermittent fasting than we would advise you not to follow it. The best way to find out if you can observe intermittent fasting is to consult with your doctor before you do any such plans, enough of that let's get into the topic of benefits.

## Weight Loss

As you know, intermittent fasting has been shown time and time again to help people lose body fat, and the keyword is body fat, as many people consider weight loss to be the key. If you're losing muscle, then there's no benefit of losing weight, as losing muscle can cause many health hazards. On the other hand, if you're losing body fat, then it could be perfect for you as it can lower the risk of many other diseases that come along. Many people who start falling intermittent fasting notice a decrease in body fat, and the reason why that is that you are not spiking your insulin all the time and converting all those carbs into fat.

As you know, when you eat anything, your insulin goes up, and if it does not have time to use up all those calories in glycogen, it will be stored into fat. The great thing about intermittent fasting is that you don't have to worry about getting all those glycogen stored into fat as you will not be eating so frequently. When you're not eating so often, then you will start burning body fat that you already have, they're for preserving your muscle while using body fat for the energy source. The great thing about that is, you will not be using any glycogen at all and merely be burning off that excess body fat.

You see, when you're intermittent fasting, your body goes into starvation mode, which is healthy for you. We have evolved to live without food for a couple of days, so it is our natural habitat not to eat food all the time. What intermittent fasting does helps us with our back in the daily routine and use body fat for energy?

## Muscle Gain

There have been many studies showing that intermittent fasting can help you put on muscle, and the truth is that intermittent fasting is perfect for putting on muscle and losing body fat. When you're intermittent fasting your body will be increasing your hormone production of growth hormone and testosterone. Especially in men, which is why intermittent fasting is the ideal scenario for natural athletes to put on muscle if you're someone who's abusing steroids then there's no benefit for you to use intermittent fasting when it comes to putting on muscle, however if use the healthy route and not use any steroids then intermittent fasting can be the answer for you. When you're intermittent fasting, your growth hormone can go up to 4000% office natural levels. As you know, growth hormone has been shown to put on and preserve muscle while increasing your bone density.

This is a no-brainer for natural athletes, as you will be increasing your testosterone and growth hormone at the same time you will put on muscle. On the other hand, you will also be cleaning out your gut, which will help you digest food a lot more efficiently. Many people don't know this, but intermittent fasting can help you clean out your stomach, having a healthy gut is very important when you're looking towards putting on muscle so make sure that you consider that when starting any muscle gaining plan.

## Mental Fog

Intermittent fasting has also been shown to reduce mental fog. As you know, mental fog can be one of the most annoying things you can face when you're trying to achieve something in your work or personal life. What intermittent fasting does is help you not worry about digesting and focus on feeding your brain. Let me explain when you're eating all the time your body concentrated on understanding the food. When you're intermittent fasting body does not have to worry about food and in fact, give you the mental focus you need. Most of the time, people cannot focus on is because they don't have the energy to concentrate as their body is digesting their food. As simple as a sound, but it's true when you're not understanding, you are a lot more focused on the work that you're doing only because your body has nothing else to do. If your organization is free of any digestion on any other thing that it has to focus on, that's when you can take up all the things you want to do so if you're going to focus a lot more and rid of the mental fog your body will facilitate that for you very directly. Also, there have been many scientific studies showing that intermittent fasting, along with ketogenic diet, can help you tremendously to focus. As you know, insulin production can help us feel a lot more lethargic, which is why when following a ketogenic diet and intermittent fasting, insulin levels won't be out of whack, and therefore, you will have a lot less mental fog and a lot more mental clarity and focus.

## Reduce Blood Pressure

As you know, intermittent fasting as shown to reduce blood pressure, which makes it an excellent plan for people to follow when it comes to putting on muscle and losing body fat. If you're eating a lot more food, which should be our goal when it comes to putting on muscle, then chances are your blood pressure will be going up.

However, when you're following intermittent fasting, that's something you don't have to worry about it, like intermittent fasting, as shown to reduce blood pressure. There have been many scientific studies showing that intermittent fasting can and will lower blood pressure, so it is one of the best things to follow when it comes to lowering your blood pressure and to see better health benefits overall. Whether it is your goal to lose fat or build muscle having a lower blood pressure is very crucial for you as well help your cardiovascular health and wellness. Cardiovascular health and wellness are essential as a house you live a long, fruitful life, so keep that into consideration when following intermittent fasting.

## Lower Cholesterol Levels

Recently there was a 3-week study showing that intermittent fasting can reduce cholesterol levels tremendously. In study showed that people reduce their bad cholesterol by a couple of points. Without getting to sign to pick on you, intermittent fasting has been scientifically proven to lower the bad cholesterol in your body. If you are facing cholesterol issues, then definitely consider intermittent fasting as a can help you with lowering cholesterol levels. Cholesterol is a silent killer in the United States, which is why it is essential to understand how cholesterol works and how it can help you or hinder you. Meaning the right amount of natural cholesterol level is essential, however when it gets too high, and it is mostly the wrong cholesterol level, then chances are that you are not in the right place when it comes to health. Which is why it is essential to understand how cholesterol levels work and how to reduce them, if you're following intermittent fasting then that's something you don't have to worry about as it does everything for you.

## Cancer

Intermittent fasting is also shown to reduce the risk of cancer. As you know, cancer grows in our body very rapidly. There have been many scientific studies showing that intermittent fasting can help us get rid of cancer once and for all. If you didn't know, there was one man who fasted for ten days Non-Stop and got rid of his disease. We don't know how accurate that is, and please don't put us on it, but this is what people have been saying about intermittent fasting and cancer. Intermittent fasting is indeed the new way to get rid of cancer, as much professional say. Having to control what you eat and when you eat it is essential, what intermittent fasting does is that it allows us to get rid of all the bad cells in our body by using a full cycle known as autophagy. Has General Auto Peggy as a process where your body gets rid of the old battery and makes new cells in your body. This is why intermittent fasting can and will reduce the risk of cancer, consider that when following intermittent fasting.

## Reduce Insulin Resistance

As you know, intermittent fasting can reduce insulin sensitivity, which is why intermittent fasting has to be followed by many people if they want to see better results. Insulin sensitivity is significant, and being insulin resistant means that you will not be digesting any food that is going into your body. Many people who have diabetes tend to be insulin resistant, controlling this hormone is very important for overall health and Longevity. What intermittent fasting does as it does not spike up your insulin randomly, what it gives you as a leveled insulin level product that will help you not only to say healthy but to help you digest food. This is very important when you're following intermittent fasting and trying to live a long healthy life; controlling this hormone wall dictates how well and how many diseases he avoids in the future. Make sure you use intermittent fasting for the right reasons, meaning taking care of your health and body. There have been many scientific studies showing that intermittent fasting will make you a lot more insulin sensitive, which is something we want as we get older; we become more insulin resistant.

## Increase Longevity

With all these benefits comes durability, we have been talking about it briefly in this chapter so far. But as you can see, intermittent fasting and definitely help you with longevity and how long you will live. Which is why periodic fasting is one of the most crucial eating plans to follow when it comes to overall health and wellness, the truth is that intermittent fasting will not only help you put on muscle and lose body fat, but it will help you to live a longer life overall. Understanding this is very important when it comes to bettering your life, you have to realize that health is not just about looking good and feeling good it is about longevity and how long you stay healthy for. What intermittent fasting provides you with a reduction of any diseases, or attracting any conditions and on top of that, giving you the health and body that you want. Intermittent fasting can indeed increase your longevity. In combination with all these benefits, intermittent fasting can genuinely help you understand what life is about. Increase longevity will give you a lot more benefits such as you get older; you will not have any health complications or minimal, on top of that you will not be taking any medications or needing any if you follow a healthful eating plan like intermittent fasting.

## DNA

Intermittent fasting has been shown to preserve your DNA and to keep it healthy, and we will not get into this topic to genuinely as it has not been backed up by science as much. However, there have been many studies showing that intermittent fasting will help you not only to fight off any hazardous issues with your DNA, but it will help you preserve it. Preserving your DNA is very important, which is why you need to follow intermittent fasting.

## Fertility

Intermittent fasting has been shown to increase productivity in men, as the hormone production goes up, so does the fertility. If you are a man looking to improve your sperm count, then there is no better way for you to go about it than to follow intermittent fasting. This will naturally increase your fertility without messing with any medications, and it is always best for you to increase your sperm count through natural means than to take any medications for it, definitely consider intermittent fasting when trying to increase sperm count or to increase fertility. Now there have been some sort of thing that intermittent fasting can increase women's fertility as well. However, we will not tell you that it does, for sure, as it has not been backed up yet.

## Cell Rejuvenation

As you know, intermittent fasting has been very well-known for autophagy, which is a cell rejuvenation process. When it comes to intermittent fasting and cell Rejuvenation, they going hand-in-hand. If you're looking to better your health and detoxify your body fully, then there's no better way to go about it later to follow intermittent fasting. Make sure that you follow intermittent fasting for the right reasons, which means that you're trying to detoxify your body inside and out. Intermittent fasting will not only detoxify your gut, but it will also detoxify yourself the way it functions everything that you can think of intermittent fasting while detoxified. The truth is that most of the time, humans are spending their time digesting their food. Therefore they get in no time to detoxify themselves. We need to detoxify your body naturally, and that comes through starvation, which is why intermittent fasting is one of the best ways to not only rejuvenate yourself but to detoxify your body.

## Detox

Now that we have extensively talked about cell Rejuvenation let's talk about detoxification and how it works and intermittent fasting. When you're fasting, your body does not have to worry about digestion, which is why it is an excellent idea for your body to start detoxifying itself. This is one of the reasons why he will feel a lot more cleaner internally when following intermittent fasting. Many people who follow intermittent fasting feel completely detox within 15 days of starting the plan.

Moreover, intermittent fasting will Detox by everything in your body that you can think about, from your nails to your hair to every single cell in your body.

Intermittent fasting is a lot more thorough than a green drink detox, which is why periodic fasting is highly recommended by not only fitness experts but doctors these days. Detoxifying your body is significant, and it is similar to getting an oil change in your car. If you want to keep your vehicle nice and to run, then you need to do regular maintenance, which includes oil change, the same thing goes with your body, which is why you need to detoxify your body as often and as thorough as you can.

## Reduce Stress and Inflammation

Intermittent fasting has shown a significant reduction in inflammation. As you know, information causes a lot of many chronic diseases such as Alzheimer's, dementia, obesity, diabetes, and much more. Now, there are many ways that intermittent fasting helps you get rid of inflammation. The first one being autophagy, as you know, intermittent fasting helps you with cell rejuvenation cleans up itself by eating out the old self and rejuvenating them with the newer, stronger ones. If your body does not rejuvenate itself with more new cells, the older ones that have stayed for an extended period can cause inflammation.

As you know, the average diet does not allow for cell rejuvenation to happen; this is where intermittent fasting comes in as it has been proven to help with the process of autophagy. Another way intermittent fasting enables you to get rid of inflammation would be by producing ketones. When your fasting your body uses up all the glycogen stores, which makes it start using stored fat for fuel, and when fats are broken down for energy, ketones are produced. One of the most popular ketones in your body will block a part of your immune system, which is responsible for inflammatory disorders. Another way intermittent fasting helps you lower the risk of inflammation is by making you insulin sensitive. When your body becomes insulin resistant, you will be holding much glucose in your bloodstream. More glucose in your blood will create inflammation, and intermittent fasting allows your body to get rid of all the glucose, which helps you reduce inflammation in your body.

Now that we've talked about many ways intermittent fasting enables you to reduce inflammation, let's talk about how intermittent fasting can help you get rid of stress. You see, inflammation and stress go hand in hand. If you have high levels of inflammation, chances are your stress levels are going to be higher. This means that if you lower your inflammation, you will reduce your stress levels, and as you know, fasting helps with better brain function. Intermittent fasting enables you to send better signals to your brain, which would equal a better functioning brain.

When your mind is functioning at its highest peak, your levels of stress dropdown, better brain function will also help you get rid of any stress you might be having, and having overall better health can help you reduce weight. Overall, all the health benefits you get from intermittent fasting will help you get rid of your stress or at least lower it. This means, even if you are not facing pressure, intermittent fasting will help you have a better functioning brain and also help you get rid of any mental fog or anxiety you might be dealing with. What that in mind, always make sure you consult a physician if you are noticing much more stress than you can handle, as it can be something severe and not fixable by intermittent fasting.

# Chapter 3: Different Types of Fasting Method

Since intermittent fasting has come out, there have been several methods which are being popularized by many fitness experts and gurus. At first, it was a simple fasting strategy, which was fast for 16 hours and eat for 8 hours. But since then, we have discovered multiple different ways of fasting, which are being used for fat loss and overall well-being.

In today's chapter, we will be talking about the seven main intermittent fasting methods, which are being used by most fitness professionals and experts out there. One of the best things in regards to following intermittent fasting is the ability to have choices. When fasting, you have so many ways to go about it that it makes it very user-friendly, as you will learn later on in this chapter. Truthfully if you are deciding to follow intermittent fasting, then you should have no excuse. Intermittent fasting works with you instead of against you, unlike most diets out there.

There are many ways to go about fasting, and we will be talking about those in this chapter. Just remember, even though you might have found the right fasting cycle for your lifestyle needs, that doesn't mean it will fit your goal. For instance, if your goal is to notice more health benefits from fast rather than weight loss, then there are some fast that works better when compared to other options. Be aware, even though all fasts will help you lose weight and live a healthier life, you still need to make sure that you are following the plan which is right for your needs.

## The 12 Hours Fast

Fasting for 12 hours is one of the ways to get started with fasting. That is the easiest way to learn how fasting works and to figure out how your body reacts to it. As I previously mentioned before, women tend to find fasting a bit more difficult because of their reproductive systems. Which makes a 12-hour fast an excellent tool for women to find out how their body reacts, and to slowly start to control their hunger cravings.

The 12-hour fast is very simple to follow, and you will be fasting for half the day and eating for half the day. When I put it like that, it doesn't sound so bad, does it?.

Although a 12-hour fast is still considered a fast and you will see some benefits from it, It won't be as drastic as something like a 16 hour fast or anything along that line. The 12-hour fast works great to get your body to prepare for more extended fasting and to show you what fasting feels like; it is merely a beginner's tool.

Nonetheless, we highly recommend 12-hour fast for women who are just starting intermittent fasting. The best way to go about 12 hours fast would be to eat from 8 am till 8 pm and then from 8 pm to 8 am not eat anything at all, even though this might sound easy for some it will still catch up on you. We recommend you follow the 12-hour fast for four weeks or until you feel like you can fast for a more extended period of time. But, most of the time, four weeks does the trick for beginners even though studies are showing that 12-hour fast tends to be the perfect time for fasting as tested on rats.

It is still recommended that you fast for a little bit of more extended time, as from personal experience and speaking with other experts in the field of intermittent fasting, they recommend ideal fast should be 16 to 20 hours. Regardless when you fast for 12 hours, you'll start to see benefits such as your insulin sensitivity going up your fat loss will kick up a notch, and you will notice more mental focus.

The 12 hour fast does everything right, which makes the 12 hours fast a jack of all trades but a master of none. It is recommended that you only follow this method for a short period to see some results, and to get used to fasting, you can pick any time frame you want to fast during. As we previously mentioned before, you can eat from 8 am to 8 pm and not eat from 8 pm to 8 am the next day. The timings won't make a drastic difference in the type of results you will be getting from the 12 hours fast. As long as you pick a time that works for you, then you should be good.

## 16 Hour Fast

This is the fasting method, which has been popularized to be intermittent fasting. Many people use this method to lose weight and to gain some muscle, especially men. But the 16 hour fast has been used successfully by women as well, Martin Bekhan, who popularized this method truly lives by it. He has noticed the better fat loss, better health, and more muscle mass by following this plan. Now, if putting on muscle is not your goal, the 16 hour fast still has some things to consider.

Most people notice when they start 16 hours fast, it is the ability to lose body fat without counting any calories or eating any specific foods. Since the 8-hour window becomes too short of overeating, followers of the 16/8 intermittent fasting method tend to see amazing results in the weight loss department. From my personal experience, I can say that 16 by eight was one of the best ways to lose fat, very easy to follow and 16 hours of fasting is not so hard, overall the results were tremendous. On top of losing weight, I noticed that my skin started to look a lot better, which was precisely what I was looking for.

In one of the newer studies done on obese individuals, they noticed not only fat loss but also reduction and blood pressure. This means the 16/8 method is excellent for fat loss and lowering the risk of cardiovascular diseases and heart diseases, even though this study was taken part in obese people it is still great to have been backed up by science. Bumping up from 12 hours to 16 hours, you will not notice a big difference in insulin sensitivity and mental focus. But, you will see more benefits towards that cellular rejuvenation and better results in fat loss.

You will also notice more detox benefits from the 16 hours fast if compared to the 12 hours, which makes the 16-hour fast a lot more similar to the 12 hours fast. Think of the 16 hours fast as the full version of intermittent fasting, whereas the 12 hour fast is the trial version, even though there is only a 4-hour difference between the two it stills makes up for a drastic change.

Once you start fasting for 16 hours instead of 12, you will notice the better fat loss and more health benefits from it. Just like the 12 hours fast, you can follow whichever way you want to pursue this fasting, the timings can be based on your lifestyle. We recommend fasting from 10 pm to 2 pm and eat from 2 pm to 10 pm, but make sure to pick a time that works for you.

## Fast for 2 Days Per Week

This fasting method was popularized by Michael Mosley, who is a doctor and journalist. Since this method has no studies to prove its benefits, it is still a method used by many people. Even though this method does not have any reliable research to back it up, benefits that are stated include better brain function, Reducing the risk of heart disease, stroke, cancer, and improving cholesterol levels.

This method can get tough to follow for some people. However, it will put you in a twenty percent calorie deficit, which is a great place to be in if your goal is to lose body fat. This could be an excellent way to lose excess body fat if you can handle it, on that note, let's talk about this method and how it works.

Also known as the 5:2 method is where the person eats an average amount of calories throughout the week and restricts their calories to five hundred/six hundred calories a day for two days. The guideline suggests five hundred calories a day for women and six hundred calories for men on fasting days. The method recommends you have two meals divided into your calories for the day when fasting, which means two meals of two fifty calories for women and two meals of three hundred calories a day for men.

Your calories will not be completely cut out throughout those two days, so make sure you are drinking a ton of water and other no-calorie liquids in between your meals on fasting days. Now the best way that you can go about using this method of fasting would generally be eating through Monday to Friday then fasting over the weekend, and my recommendation would be fast when you don't have work or if you are doing anything physically demanding like working out.

This will ensure you don't feel tired or worst go hypoglycemic as you will be "fasting" for a long time, so make sure you are fasting on days you are not working or doing anything physically demanding. Also, the great thing about this method is that there is no food restriction during non-fasting days, which is a good thing for some you foodies out there. Now there are some benefits to these methods, and let us talk about that.

The primary benefit is that you will lose body fat and that too quite quickly, as a result of eating so little during those two days of fasting. I have personally followed this plan just as an experiment, and I have to say, and I did lose body fat in those two weeks, which I followed it. If your goal is fat loss without restricting your diet as much, then this method can be the one for you.

Another benefit claimed are; lowers cholesterol, lowers the risk of heart disease and cancer, which is fantastic for everyone following this method of fasting. But then again, these benefits are claimed, not proven, so don't follow this method if your goal is to lower the risk of diseases there are other fasting methods in this book that you can follow to get those benefits. The great thing about this fasting method is that you will get to eat what you want to eat, no need to restrict yourself on non-fasting days, but if I were you, I would still be careful. Not to overeat if your goal is to lose body fat, so those are the benefits now let's talk about the cons.

This method is not the best by any means, there are some flaws to this method, and one of them was used in a positive, but it is being used in con. In this method, you can eat whatever you want to eat, which is a flaw since people will eat a ton of junk food as an excuse and not do any justice to their health. I believe that fasting should be accompanied by a well-balanced, healthy diet and having junk food on occasion, so I don't like the fact of having whatever you want on your non-fasting days as it can take away from the benefits of fasting.

Another flaw of this method is that it can be tough for some people to make it a lifestyle as fasting for two days straight can be a problem, but if it works for you, then go for it. The main flaw is that there so no backing up the claims that this method is claiming. Although this is a fasting method and fasting has a lot of benefits that have been backed up, this method doesn't, so as I said before, don't follow this diet if your sole purpose is to lower the risk of diseases. If you follow a workout plan that requires strength training, then this fasting method might not be the one for you, as this method can hinder your workout quality as it did for some people.

So now you know all about the 5:2 method, this method can be used with great success if your goal is to lose body fat and have no restrictions on your diet on non - fasting days. But please use this method for the right reasons, don't use it if you want a lowered risk of diseases as studies have not proved it.

Other fasting methods can be followed if your goal is lower the risks, and if your goal is to get stronger and put on some muscle, then this method won't be ideal as this method can affect your workouts. All in all, if this method is being used for the right reasons, then it can lead you to great success in weight loss goals. If this method matches your lifestyle and goals, then follow this fasting protocol. But our recommendation would be to use this plan with a grain of salt and to only use it for a short period. As we don't think this method is a sustainable fasting protocol like the 16/8.

# Alternate Day Fasting

Very similar to the two days a week fasting, this method requires you usually eat on one day and the next day fast. For the fasting period, you are allowed to have 500 calories a day for women and 600 calories for men. However, you can take it up a notch and not eat any calories at all, which is not recommended by most but done by some. The whole reason behind the alternative fasting was to help people lose weight quickly; people have seen similar results as the 5:2 method, where they lose a lot of body fat fast. This method has also been shown to lower the risk of diabetes, which is a great plus for people looking to lose weight and reduces the risk of diabetes.

This method allows you typically to fast three days in a week, putting you at a 25% caloric deficit, which is a little bit more than the 5:2 method. What I like about this fasting method is the frequency. If compared to the 5:2 method, you are fasting more frequently and more regularly. Whereas in the 5:2 method, you are eating whatever you want for five days, and then fasting for two whole days straight, this makes it a little bit more reputable for me.

That being said, the same cons follow for this one. On your fasting days, you aren't genuinely fasting, and you can if you decide to, but it not healthy, especially for women to fast for 24 hours so frequently. Another disadvantage of this diet would be the allowance of eating whatever they want, although it is excellent for people who like to eat junk food, it is not so healthy, especially on fasting days. Most people will eat something non-dense like a slice of pizza, whereas you should be eating more of a dense meal to see better health changes overall.

Which makes this diet an excellent tool for weight loss, since it will help keep in a caloric deficit throughout the week. However, this diet is not a great way to see some health benefits, making it very similar to the 5:2 fasting method. One great thing about this method, when compared to the 5:2 method, is the ability to maintain strength during workouts. Since your fast will be very cyclical, your chances of losing a lot of strength will be lower, which makes this diet ideal for someone looking to lose fat and maintain a healthy strength level throughout.

Finally, make sure that if you decide to follow this fasting protocol, it is for the right reasons. If you want to lose weight quickly and you have a comfortable going lifestyle, then this plan might be the answer for you. Also, just like the 5:2 method, I would not recommend you follow this fasting method for a prolonged period as it can be unhealthy. However, besides all the negatives of this fasting protocol, there are a ton of positives, especially if you are looking to lose weight.

## Weekly 24 Hour Fast

The 24 hour fast has been used widely by many fitness professionals out there. Brad Pilon, the author of eat stop eat once, said: "prolonged calorie restriction is the only way to fat loss." This is the reason why the weekly 24 hours fast was created, easy as it sounds once a week you eat no calories. After you have completed the fast, eat regularly as you would if you were not fasting.

The whole premises behind this fasting protocol is to put you in a caloric deficit. For example, if you require 2,500 calories to maintain your weight, then eat 2,500 calories a day but fast for one of those days. The claims of the weekly fasting method are, weight loss lowered the risk of diseases such as diabetes and many others. Unfortunately, in the weekly 24 hours fasts, the claims haven't been backed up with science. However, this fasting protocol has shown to speed up weight loss.

Many followers of this fasting protocol have seen fantastic weight loss effects, which makes this a tremendous tool for fat loss, also really good for detoxing your body. The 24-hour fast will help you get rid of any toxins in your intestines and other organs, believe it or not digesting food is a hard task for our body. Not giving your intestines and other organs a break from digesting can lead to poor digestion, this is where the weekly 24-hour fasting shines. People who follow this fast, have noticed better digestion and healthier hair and skin because of cell rejuvenation effects it has.

The weekly 24 hours fast has shown to help with cell rejuvenation or also known as autophagy, which makes this protocol great for followers looking to lose weight and see results like better digestion and cell rejuvenation. Even though this protocol comes with a host of benefits, there are still some concerns. Even though you are fasting for only one day a week, 24 hours fast can become very hard for some, especially women, because of the hunger craving.

It would be best if you had a great support system to pull through the 24 hours fast; another falls back of this fast would be the post-binge eating cravings. Many followers have noticed insane amounts of food craving the day after fasting if you overeat throughout the week and fast for only one day, the chances of you losing weight will be slim to none. Make sure you have the will power to avoid these food cravings once you get them, as indulging in them would not be great if you are looking to lose body fat.

In conclusion, this protocol is ideal for people who have fasted for an extended period before. We would not recommend this fasting protocol to an absolute beginner, as it can be tough to follow through. Fasting has no benefit if you can't follow thru, so make sure you pick the right one.

## Meal Skipping

This method is something people used to their body prepared for fasting, now to be clear, I don't consider this to be as beneficial as most fasting protocol, and I repeat I don't believe this method to be as helpful as most fasting protocol. Now saying that would I recommend this method to someone else? The answer is yes! Why you ask, the simple reason this method is one of the easiest to follow, and it prepares you for fasting purposes that will help you with better physical health and wellness. Would I recommend someone make this method their lifestyle, and the answer would be no.

Only consider this if you have never followed a fasting method before, and you want to slowly build up to a longer fast, which would make this method the one for you. Some readers can completely ignore this method and start with other fasting methods listed above if you have experience fasting before for fifteen days, then you should be able to follow a more "intense" protocols. None the less, let's talk about this method. The whole point of this method is for you to start skipping meals, in between the day to ease you into a longer fast.

So what you can do if you decide to follow this plan is to start by skipping breakfast then have some lunch and dinner, slowly building up to a longer fast. If you want, you can even have a snack instead of skipping breakfast, which will make it easier for you. The whole point is to make you feel comfortable before taking the big step, and this method allows you to take baby steps into the vast realm of fasting. Which I think is the plus of this fasting method.

There are some benefits to this type of fasting method. One of the things that you might notice, especially starting, is that you will most likely lose some fat. Often we don't realize how much we overeat, and the average person tends to eat more than he or she should. Most North American diet consists of foods that are loaded with carbohydrates, sugar, and a ton of "bad fat" such as trans-fat in their diet, which leads to most of the obesity issues in our society. One meal, on average, tends to be six hundred to a thousand calories per meal.

Now if you skip one meal every day for a week, you are looking to cut about forty two-hundred to seven thousand calories a week, a pound of fat has thirty-five-hundred calories so you can defiantly see some fat loss benefits. This method will also give your gut a break from digesting all this processed food that some readers might be eating, which means better gut health overall. You can see all the benefits of this method, but this fasting method is something that you should not use as a protocol to lose fat in the long term as it can leave you malnourished in the end.

See our primary goal with this book is to show you how to live a healthy life both physically and mentally, sometimes our body gives us signals to skip meals and without even knowing you would skip a meal just because you felt like it. We are always using this method, but then the next day instead of three, we have four meals and not to mention a big and unhealthy one. So our body always makes us clean our gut time to time organically, one thing people can get carried away within this method is since they skip a meal they think they can have anything their heart desires.

This should not be the case, in my opinion, you need to be eating healthy doesn't matter if you choose to fast or not if you want to be free of health complications in the future and looking good. By eating healthy, we make sure to get all our micronutrients in, like our vitamins and minerals for the day and your macronutrients like your calories, fats, carbs, and protein, depending on your fitness and aesthetic goals.

Another thing that should not be left out is the consumption of water if you can't seem to skip the meal, and you tend to get hungry, drink more water during your fast. Not only will that hydrate you, but it will also get rid of toxins in your body and help you with fat loss if that's your goal. At the end of the day, if you want to ease into this fasting lifestyle, you should use this method as a tool to get you up to a longer fast, so you don't fall off track. Just make sure you are using it for the right reasons if 12 hours soon is too much for you to begin with, then consider this protocol and move up from there.

## The Warrior Diet

This method is more based on our ancestor's eating habits, created by Ori Hofmekler. This method suggests us to "eat like a warrior." In the earlier times, fasting thru out the day and only having a four-hour window to eat a big meal was a norm for us humans, as Hofmekler thinks humans were created to eat like this. This method was based on his belief system and how humans should be eating instead of using science-based evidence and studies. In this method, you are allowed to have mostly whatever you want in that four-hour eating window, go by what you feel, and also don't go by macronutrient count eat how much ever you want to eat.

Another thing which is advocated in this method is that you will be more suited for burning fat for energy, claimed by Ori Hofmekler. If you follow this diet, you will lose body fat and won't have to count calories. So in this method, you have to fast for twenty hours and have an eating window of only four hours.

Now, if you are currently using the "16/8" method, then switching up to the warrior diet won't be such a shock to your body, but if you are going to go from an average eating habit to this, then I will be hard for you physically. I would recommend starting with fasting for twelve hours and slowly building up to the twenty-hour mark. If fasting for twelve hours can get challenging for you, then I would suggest slowly skipping meals like breakfast, and then when that feels easy, slowly skipping breakfast and lunch until you get to the point where you can fast for twenty hours of the day.

Now, the way it recommends to follow this method is to fast in the day time and eat at the night time, as warriors would do after hunting and preparing their meals at the end of the day. You can have your meals at any time even before going to bed, and this diet should be followed just like the ancient times like the warrior did, meaning fast in the morning and feast at night. In this diet, you can have fruits and vegetables, but it recommended you stay away from canned fruits and vegetables, also their juices.

In this method, it's highly recommended to workout in an empty stomach to stimulate a warrior lifestyle. It is suggested to work out for thirty to forty-five minutes of intense workouts, with the use of compound movements like pull-ups, push-ups, and squats, which use more than one muscle group. You can still consume water and other non-calorie drinks, so don't be scared to workout, not hydrated.

So, in conclusion, this diet is based on a lifestyle that warriors had back in ancient times, which was a selling factor for some people, including me. Since this diet has no science or studies to back it up, it can be a turn off to some people when it comes to following a fasting protocol since they might want to see health benefits like lowering the risk of diabetes and other things of that nature.

Even though this method is quite similar to "16/8", I think it should help lower the risk of diseases but then again no research on it. On the other hand, if your goal is to feel and look like a warrior, this method will be the right one for you. Although I haven't followed this plan long enough to see drastic physical changes, I have met people who have completely transformed their physical appearance and health; also their energy levels have drastically changed for the better. This method has resulted in success for most people, and when I followed it for one week, I felt like "16-8" is ideal for me as I was feeling the same on this method.

One thing I didn't like about this method is that you have to work out on an empty stomach, as with "16/8," I would workout fed. So if you don't mind working out on an empty stomach and you want to live a warrior lifestyle, then this method might be for you.

Even though this goes with no saying, always get recommended by your doctor before you follow this method or another method listed in this book. This method can be pretty hard for you in the beginning; make sure you don't go into it without easing into fasting. I hope you see the results that you are looking for following this fasting method.

We have now gone through all the fasting methods, and you might have learned a lot from this chapter. Many people might say that fasting works differently on men as compared to women, but besides the hunger portion, it is the same. As long as you follow these fasts safety and with the guidance of your doctor, you should be fine.

Also, if you read these chapters carefully, you might have noticed that some fasts are suited better for specific results. Even though all fasts will help you achieve fat loss and overall health benefits, there are some protocols tailored for weight loss and others which are suited for whole, healthy well-being.

When you are picking out which fasting protocol to follow, consider lifestyle, and your goals as most of them will fit your needs. Overall know what you want out of intermittent fasting. Also, if you pick the right fasting protocol, then you should see the benefits which you have been looking to get.

# Chapter 4: Intermittent Fasting and Who Can Do It

As we mentioned to you previously, intermittent fasting does not yield drastically different results in both men and women. However, there are many differences in regard to how women should follow intermittent fasting. The great news is that women can take part in all the fast's listed in this book, regardless we need to talk about intermittent fasting for women. Also, it is a definite no if you are pregnant for you to start fasting.

Some claims are suggesting that intermittent fasting needs to be modified, which is true to a certain degree if women use the easier going fasting protocols, which are available to review in the previous chapters. Then they should have no problem with intermittent fasting, and the problems start to occur when 48 hours+ fasts begin to take place.

Nonetheless, you should know the claims and studies done on women in regard to intermittent fasting. There was one study suggesting that blood sugar worsened in women after three weeks of intermittent fasting. Moreover, many sources are claiming that changes in women's menstrual cycle will occur. As we explained before, because of the woman's reproductive system, they are susceptible to lower calories.

Hence, making people believe that women do not indulge in intermittent fasting, which we don't agree with. If done tastefully, intermittent fasting has resulted in excellent health and weight loss benefits for women. So in this chapter, we will go thru exactly how intermittent fasting affects women in all aspects, such as hormones, hunger craving, and many more things are on the agenda. With that in mind, let's get into the nitty-gritty.

## The Key to Intermittent Fasting for Women in Autophagy

You might have heard of autophagy in this book so far, now let me explain to you what autophagy truly means. Autophagy is a biological process that comes from the Greek word "auto," meaning "self" and "phagy" meaning "eat." It is a process where our body cleans out the bad cells and replace them with newer healthy ones, which is excellent for anyone looking to live a healthier life.

But sometimes, our body cannot get this process going for hosts of reasons. Mainly because we eat the food we can't digest properly, which makes our body work extra hard to cope up with the food instead of getting rid of "bad cells." As we get older, the process becomes less efficient. One of the proven ways to fix this issue, especially for women, is by fasting for 12 or more hours and allowing your body to focus more on getting rid of the "bad cells" by replacing them with newer and stronger ones.

This method works exceptionally well, especially on women, to rejuvenate their cells and to see the health benefits. The great news about autophagy is that you don't need to fast for an indefinite amount of time to notice the results, 12 to 16 hours of fast will do. This means women don't need to put yourself at risk by fasting for a prolonged period; this makes intermittent fasting a tool for women looking to stay young for more extended periods.

Remember that autophagy should not be just for anti-aging purposes, as it can help you with hosts of things. Consider autophagy as a detox for your whole body, and believe it or not; most people need it. Forget cleansing diets, and if you truly want to detox your body, then you need to fast for at least 12 hours a day.

For women, 12-16 hours should not result in adverse effects. You will also reduce the risk of cancer because you will have newer and stronger cells at your disposal; another great benefit would be the fact that your metabolism will go up helping you with weight loss.

All in all, promoting the process of autophagy a great way to encourage better health, especially for women. Having healthier cells in a women's body will help you by having a better reproductive system, and you will have a higher chance of conceiving. Even though these claims haven't been backed up, it is still good to know that some excellent benefits come with intermittent fasting for women.

Finally, you will notice benefits such as better skin, better digestion of more energy throughout the day. To see the best results, fast for 12 to 16 hours a day, three times a week. Make sure you space out your days, instead of doing all the fasts back to back. If you want to fast through the week as many do, then make sure not to prolong it for more than 6-8 weeks.

# Fasting and Female Hormones

Intermittent fasting has shown to affect females' hormones, and there are some things women need to consider before they start fasting. Some studies are showing how intermittent fasting can negatively impact the female's reproductive system, and the reason why these shifts occur is that women are sensitive to lower calorie intake. When the calories are low for women, a small part of the brain known as the hypothalamus is affected.

Hypothalamus can disrupt the production of gonadotropin-releasing hormone (GnRH), which is responsible for releasing the two reproductive hormones, luteinizing hormone (LH) and follicle-stimulating hormone (FSH). Once these hormones have been affected negatively from an extended period by restricting calories, you will be running a risk of irregular periods, infertility, poor bone health, and other health risks. Even though autophagy has shown to do the opposite, it puts women in a complicated situation when it comes to fasting. For that reason, we don't recommend women fast for more than 24 hours as it can affect women's hormones in a very drastic manner.

Instead, women should use a modified approach that we talked about in this book. To make sure women don't notice any hormone imbalance, fast alternate days instead of back to back, keeping you in a safe place. If you want to fast aggressively for weight loss, then our recommendation is not to prolong it for more than 4-6 weeks. But then again, make sure you consult a professional before you may start fasting as everybody is different. On the plus side, there are many benefits women will notice if they begin fasting the right way. As we know, heart disease is killing people every day, in one study done on obese women showed that intermittent fasting lowered LDL cholesterol or which is the leading cause of heart problems in North America.

Also, intermittent fasting has shown to make you more insulin sensitive. In one study of 100 obese women showed that six months of intermittent fasting reduced insulin levels by 29% and insulin resistance by 19 %, although blood sugar remained the same. Having higher sensitively to insulin has shown to lower the risk of type 2 diabetes, but intermittent fasting may not be beneficial for women as it is for men in regards to blood sugar. In mice, it has been shown to increase longevity by 33%, although long term studies on humans are yet to be determined.

Finally, intermittent fasting can reduce inflammation levels. Even though more studies need to be executed for women and intermittent fasting, it is pretty clear that there are hosts of benefits if done right. As long as you are taking intermittent fasting the right way, and you are not abusing it, your hormones should be in check. Remember, if you are pregnant, this might affect you very differently. Moreover, we do not recommend women fast when they are pregnant or trying to conceive, but as long as you know the repercussions of fasting too long.

## Why Intermittent Fasting Effects Women's Hormone More Than Men's?

If you have been doing research online, then you might have read claims such as "intermittent fasting is not for women" or "if women intermittent fast, their hormones will be out of whack." This isn't the case, as we will discuss how intermittent fasting truly affects women's hormone as when compared to men.

To briefly talk about men, they were created to "hunt and gather" so to speak. Unlike women, they do not have to carry a baby, which is one of the reasons why intermittent fasting does not affect men as drastically as women. Women are more susceptive to hormones that are related to hunger, and the reason behind is women's reproductive system, as previously mentioned.

The good news is, it will not affect your thyroid as some "experts" will claim, women recognize hunger at a higher degree than men. We recently talked about the Hypothalamus gonadotropin-releasing hormone (GnRH), luteinizing hormone (LH), and follicle-stimulating hormone (FSH), which is responsible for making testosterone and sperm in men and triggering estrogen and ovulation in women.

Women tend to trigger these hormones differently when compared to men, and the main problem occurs because of kisspeptin. For readers that don't know what kisspeptin is, it is a protein-like molecules that neurons use to communicate with each other. Women tend to produce more kisspeptin when compared to men, which is a precursor to (GnRH).

As you know (GnRH) is going to dictate how women produce estrogen and how men are going to produce testosterone, another thing is that kisspeptin is very sensitive to the hunger hormone. If you remember, we mentioned that women are more vulnerable to the hunger hormone when compared to men? The reason behind this is kisspeptin, which causes women to produce less kisspeptin and leads to lower progesterone. One study done on rats showed that when female rats fast for one day, which is more like a week for women, it caused them to lose 19% of their body weight, but their ovaries shrunk significantly.

Also, they noticed that female rats luteinizing hormone plummeted, and their estrogen levels went through the roof. To briefly touch upon thyroid, t3 levels were deceased. But, t3 levels are always decreasing between meals. The t4, which is responsible for producing thyroid, remained the same, which means the thyroid isn't being affected drastically. It is always suggested that you get regular blood work done to ensure your thyroid is fine, but one of them to tell if it isn't is by seeing how could you get.

If you feel cold all the time, then the chances are your thyroid is lower. If you notice that you are getting starving throughout the day, and it becomes tough to fast, then break the fast and try it again later. As a woman, you need to listen to your more than men, as women tend to be more sensitive to hormones when intermittent fasting.

## Eating Enough Calories

Since you now know the science behind intermittent fasting and how it can affect women's hormones, let us talk about eating enough calories, especially for women. Believe it or not, this is an important topic to discuss. Especially for women who are much more sensitive to hunger hormones or hormones in general when compared to men. Even though you might be fasting for weight loss, it is critical that you enough calories support your bodily function as a woman. Ideally speaking, women who are trying to lose weight should not eat bellow 200 calories of their maintenance, calculating your maintenance calories the formula is (bodyweight x 12).

Meaning, if your maintenance calories are 2,000 and you are looking to lose weight, then you should not cut it down less than 1,800. If you are someone looking to lose weight with intermittent fasting, we recommend having a macronutrients break down of 20% carbs 50% protein and 30% fats. This shows the percentage of calories coming from specific macronutrients.

We are keeping the carbs low to prevent insulin spikes in check. If you are looking to lose weight, we want to keep the insulin as flatlined as possible. However, if you are someone looking to maintain weight and reap the health benefits of intermittent fasting, then we recommend having a macronutrient breakdown of 30% carbs 40% protein 30% fats since we have covered the calorie intake, lets briefly talk about the types of food you should be eating. What you eat to break your fast is just as essential as the number of calories you should be consuming. One thing you need to understand is not going overboard on the fasting.

As you know, carbs tend to spike your insulin, and when you're fasting, your insulin levels are low, meaning whatever you eat, your body will be sensitive to it. Having spikes of insulin slows down fat loss. Therefore lower insulin equals more fat burning. If you break your fast with higher amounts of carbs, you will be shutting down the fat burning process. Instead, what we recommend is eating two meals when you break into your eating window. The first one should be lower in carbs and higher in fats and protein; this will ensure you don't turn off your fat burning and get the most out of your fast. The second meal could be higher carbs, and this will help you get ready for the next day if you are fasting.

Another to remember is that your gut will be susceptible to high acidic foods such and drinks, so make sure you stick to foods that are less acidic when you break your fast. Greek yogurt, chicken with some veggies, or even soup works great to break your fast. Now whether your goal is to lose weight or live a healthier life, it is essential that you follow the right calorie intake and macronutrient intake. These tips will go a long way with both the criteria listed.

## How to Avoid Feeling Underfed

Since you now know how much to eat, let's talk about how to prevent feeling underfed. Believe it or not, both men and women notice this problem, which causes them to overeat. We need to make sure you don't feed underfed to avoid things like breaking a fast too soon or overeating. There is a couple of technique we can provide you with that shall help you with the feeling of underfed.

The first technique we recommend would be eating wholesome, healthy foods that have a lot of fiber in them. Even though you are free to eat whatever you want, it is still not recommended that you eat unhealthily. When you break you're fast, the food you should be eating is high fiber lower carbs and moderate protein. What the fiber will do is help you feel fuller throughout the day, making you feel less underfed.

An example of this would be to eat more green leafy vegetables, as they will make you feel fuller for a long time. Since we are on the topic of plants, let us talk about vitamins, you need to have micronutrients dense meals when you are fasting. If you are feeling underfed when fasting, the chances are that you are not consuming enough vitamins and minerals, making you feel underfed.

Make sure you are getting your daily mineral intake during your eating window to avoid such adverse effects, you could take a vitamin supplement during your fasting window to obtain your minerals. But don't use the supplement to take care of your vitamin needs, make sure you are eating healthy foods instead of junk food to feel thoroughly fed. Also, drinking water for the whole day is essential. If you are not drinking enough water, then you have a much higher chance of feeling underfed.

Not only will the water help you feel fuller, but it will also help you to get rid of toxins in your body. Water is a must for a better fasting experience; another thing which can curb your hunger is coffee. If you drink black coffee during your fast, it will help you control any hunger cravings you might be having, which will make you feel less underfed.

One recommendation would be drinking your coffee during the earlier times of the day, instead of later. As drinking coffee then makes you crash pretty hard, which will make you crave more, so make sure you stay away from coffee later during the day. Perhaps consume your coffee earlier in the morning or before your workout works the best, but the main take away would be not to consume junk. Even though fasting allows you to eat whatever you want, it doesn't mean you should, as it can lead you feeling underfed and hungry in the long run. Make sure you are following all these steps to ensure not handling underfed, and as you know, women tend to experience more hunger.

## How Often Should Women Follow Intermittent Fasting

When it comes to fasting, women are more sensitive than men. Hence, making the timings and the duration of fasting a bit more restricted than men. Experts suggest that women should have a more relaxed approach than men. This may include shorter fasting days, lesser fasting days, and sometimes eating some food during the fast. We always recommend women to not fast longer than 24 hours, that's why all the fasting protocols listed in this book have a fasting window of no more than 24 hours.

Also, whichever fasting protocol you decide to choose, make sure it is sustainable to you. As it can lead to fewer results overall and disappointment, these being the surface level issues. If women fast for longer than 24 hours, it can lead to hormones going out of whack, and you what could happen then. Another thing to make sure of would be to fast consecutive days in the beginning, and it is recommended that women fast three times a week on consecutive days to ensure they can handle it.

Follow this protocol for the first three weeks, and eventually, if your physician gives you the go, then start lasting longer. With that being said, some women should not follow intermittent fasting. If you are pregnant, trying to conceive, nursing, or under chronic stress, then fasting should not be done. This now brings me to the period women should fast for. Ideally, women should follow a fasting protocol for no longer than eight weeks.

It is ideal for women to take a break from internment fasting after fasting for eight weeks, women should take a whole week off from fasting ideally two weeks off. If you start to notice symptoms such as irregular periods, metabolic stress, anxiety, depression, and insomnia, then stop fasting right away and speak with your doctor. These could be a sign of fasting for too long, so make sure you are looking out for these symptoms every time. There are some fasts you should not do for a prolonged period, such as the 5:2 method and the alternate-day fasting.

These two fasting protocols make sure you are not exceeding the six-week mark of following it. Finally, women need to stay on alert when they are fasting, know your body, and make sure you feel right and healthy when you are fasting. Some hunger cravings are fine, but if you start to notice insanity high food cravings which you can't control no matter what, then it is safer to eat some food rather than put your hormones and body in danger.

Fasting can be very fragile in terms of improving health or deteriorating it, especially in women. Which means you need to make sure you ease into fasting and to take regular breaks from it. The timelines we recommend in this chapter works for most women, but consult with a professional before you start or stop a fasting protocol! Good luck.

## Symptoms You Should Lookout For

There are many signs to look for when intermittent fasting since you know most of the things related to intermittent fasting by now; let's talk about the significant symptoms to lookout. The first one being hunger, many followers of intermittent fasting will notice insane amounts of desire when following intermittent fasting. Which is a given, since you will be going from eating four to six meals throughout the day to none.

The first couple of days will require a ton of willpower to get thru, but eventually, it will subside and get better in a week. Give it some time for your body to get used to intermittent fasting, and be aware of the fact that it will be a shock in the beginning. Besides hunger, cravings for food are very evident when following intermittent fasting. Chances of you breaking your fast will be very high, especially when you are just getting started with it. You will crave foods like a candy bar, fruits, soda's anything which will give you a ton of sugar quickly. You will have to fight these cravings as they will kick in so make sure you don't indulge in them, Headaches is another thing which beginners might notice.

When you start your intermittent fasting, you will see symptoms such as headaches, don't get worried as they will subside in a week in most cases. Make sure you are drinking plenty of water during your fasting window and after, as this will make it easy for your body to cope with the headaches.

One of the main symptoms you should be looking out for would be feeling cold. You will be contacting cold for the first week, but if it continues past the three-week mark, then consider modifying your fasting protocol. Intermittent fasting has shown to increase blood flow to your fat stores for your body to use it for energy, but if you start feeling cold shivering past the three-week mark, then it is a symptom you should be looking out.

Since you will be drinking a lot of water, this will make you feel even colder throughout the day, so unless you feel cold, don't take it seriously. Speaking of drinking water, you will also notice you going to the bathroom a lot. It is because of your water consumption, and there isn't a way around it since we don't recommend you drink less water. These are the main symptoms you will notice when you first start intermittent fasting, and they usually last three weeks.

If you experience these symptoms at the same magnitude as you were the first week, then please modify your fasting protocol as it might not be suitable for your body. If you healthily want to follow intermittent fasting, then it is best to look out for these symptoms and to listen to your body. If you're going to avoid these symptoms, then ease into intermittent fasting and making sure it isn't a shock for your body from the get-go.

## Tips for Intermittent Fasting for Women

Let's talk about some quick tips women need to consider before they start intermittent fasting, as there are some great ones to find before you start. The first tip would be to drink a ton of water when fasting, pretty easy to follow and understand. You need to drink water to curb your cravings, as you know, women tend to crave foods more than men do only because of the hormone response.

Drinking water will also help you control the headache symptoms you might get, overall drinking water is a must. Drinking tea and coffee will help you manage your hunger throughout the day; it will also give you more energy in the beginning stages of fasting.

Just make sure you drink black coffee or black/green tea, don't add any sugar or milk as it will break your fast if you do that. If you find yourself around people who aren't supportive of your fasting endeavors, then make sure you stay away from them or at least avoid talking about fasting. The last thing you want is unsupportive people when you are following intermittent fasting, so make sure you stay away from them and stay positive. Finally, give yourself at least a month when you start intermittent fasting.

Many people don't realize that it will take some time to start seeing changes in their body; four weeks is a good time for your body to begin adapting to intermittent fasting. Meaning, you need to keep up the fast for at least a month for you to make a judgment whether fasting is for you or not, and most of the time, it works out in your favor. In the first four weeks of fasting, you will notice hunger waves avoid them by drinking coffee or tea. The main tip when intermittent fasting would be to not binge eat; when you break your fast, you will have the craving to binge eat.

Avoid it, follow our macros and eating patterns, which we have listed above in this chapter. If you want to develop your eating pattern, that's fine as well, make sure not a lot of carbs are on your plate in your first meal as this will make you binge eat later. Making sure you don't overeat is essential for intermittent fasting, as it will dictate your goals. If you are looking to lose weight, then make sure you eat portion-controlled meals instead of eating whatever your heart desires. These are all the primary tips, make sure you follow them, so you don't end up giving up too soon.

All in all, these tips will help you in the future. As you will see, how much easier fasting becomes for you once you start considering these tips, but don't forget to listen to your body as we previously mentioned. Looking out for your health first is very important, so if you feel like these tips are not helping you within three weeks, then modify your fasting.

# Chapter 5: Hormones

Intermittent fasting has been known to affect the body in a drastic manner, mostly in a positive manner, when done correctly. In this chapter, we will get into the specifics of it all, and also show you how intermittent fasting truly affects your body inside and out.

## Intermittent Fasting and Your Metabolism

Intermittent fasting has shown to raise your metabolism and has also proved to lower your metabolism, which is why you need to follow intermittent fasting the right way. Here's the thing when following intermittent fasting, you will most likely boost your metabolism in the beginning, as your body will go into starvation mode it will start to use your body fat for energy. Once it starts using the body fat for energy, it will have to increase metabolism. Whenever your metabolism is increased, you will be burning more calories as we know this.

However, if you keep on with intermittent fasting for a prolonged period, your body will understand and will burn calories at a much lower rate. The reason why is because your body is brilliant; it does not want to burn up many calories when it knows that there aren't back in time soon. Hence, it slows down the process of burning calories and raising metabolism. For you to get the most benefits out of intermittent fasting, you have to become smarter, more specifically, to become more intelligent than your body. The way to do that is by cycling off intermittent fasting. You will see significant fat loss benefits from intermittent fasting for about 4 to 6 weeks, after that it will go downhill. Your goal should be to cycle on and off of intermittent fasting, and this will allow you to see all the benefits while not harming your metabolism.

## How Fasting Can Hurt Your Metabolism

As we just briefly explained to you how intermittent fasting affects your metabolism, let's talk about how it can damage your metabolism when looking at the science. When your following intermittent fasting, you put yourself into a starvation mode. Once you're in starvation mode, your body will do anything possible to survive, which means burning off any glycogen in the bloodstream and start using fat stores for energy. In order to use fat stores for energy, your body will need to increase metabolism and therefore allow you to burn more fat.

Your metabolism and the number of calories you burn go hand-in-hand, which is why having high metabolism helps you burn a lot more calories. However, the thing is, your body will get used to the starvation mode and will burn a lot fewer calories once you get into it a little bit deeper. Your body is brilliant; it will only use the number of calories it needs to survive. Once it becomes acquainted with the starvation mode you put in your body in, it will become a lot more effective at burning calories and therefore lower your metabolism. If you don't follow intermittent fasting the right way, it can lead to metabolism slowing down for the rest of your life. Make sure you're following intermittent fasting the right way, and by cycling on and off.

## Fasting and Brain

Many CEOs and successful people follow intermittent fasting because of the effects it has on the brain. Even though it has not been scientifically proven, intermittent fasting has shown to increase brain function, allowing you to have more focus throughout the day to get the work done. When you're intermittent fasting, your body becomes a lot more focused because it feels like it needs to be hunting in order to get more food.

Which is simply the Primal inmate in us; when you're hunting, you need to be focused in order to get the kill, which is why when you're in the starvation mode, you become a lot more focused. From personal experience, I can tell you that intermittent fasting is helping my mental function and focus while doing anything, even driving a car while intermittent fasting has made me a lot more focus on the road.

The hormone which is released while you are intermittent fasting is known as your adrenaline hormone. Your adrenaline is a lot higher when intermittent fasting when your adrenaline is high; you're in a flight or fight situation. This is when your body will do anything possible to make sure that you're focused and do what you have to do. The adrenal hormone was more used by our ancestors not to get killed by predators. In the modern-day, we use hormone for work-related stuff or anything which requires mental focus.

## Burns Fat for Fuel

You will burn a lot more calories following intermittent fasting than you would following any diet out there. Most diets out there, make you eat 5 to 6 times a day every

2 to 3 hours. The reason why it won't work is that your glycogen will always be full, and therefore, your body will be using glycogen for energy and not be using its fat store. Here's the thing your body needs to be in the starvation mode in order to use fat stores, but your body is very smart; it will not use body fat stores if it does not need to.

What intermittent fasting does as I said is put you into starvation mode, once you're in starvation mode your body will use the fat for energy. Once your body starts using fat for energy, it will burn off the fat stores that you have, giving you a more aesthetically pleasing physique. The reason why your body will be using the fat stored glycogen is because you will not be providing your body glycogen for a long time, when you don't give your body glycogen for an extended period of time the only way it will function properly is to use the fat stores that you have in your body.

Another reason why intermittent fasting helps you burn more fat is that a puts you into ketosis. This is when your body will strictly use fat for energy and not glycogen. In later chapters, we will talk about how specific diets can help you burn more fat while following intermittent fasting. However, for now, know that intermittent fasting will help you burn more fat than glycogen throughout the day.

## Boost Your Energy

Remember how we said intermittent fasting boosts your adrenaline, which is one of the reasons why you will have more energy while intermittent fasting. When you have high amounts of adrenaline and your body, you will have more energy to do physical and mental tasks. Another way intermittent fasting helps you boost your energy is by not giving you any ups and downs in your insulin level.

Have you ever had the feeling of overeating food and feeling very tired right after, the reason why I feel exhausted right after is that your insulin is spiking up to digest their food. When your insulin spikes up, you'll feel lethargy and tiredness. When intermittent fasting, you will have no insulin spikes during your fast, which will allow you to have a sustained amount of energy throughout the day and therefore boosting power. These two things in combination will help your energy tremendously while intermittent fasting. This is why intermittent fasting raises your energy, and when you mix it up with working out, then you are set on the part of excellent energy levels throughout the day.

## Boost HGH Level

Intermittent fasting has shown to increase human growth hormone levels tremendously; let's get into the science of how this works. When you're intermittent fasting, your body will not be producing insulin or spiking sporadically throughout the day. Which is one of the reasons why your human growth hormone will go up.

The thing is growth hormone, and Insulin cannot coexist, technically they can, but if your insulin is spiking up your growth hormone will be going down and vice versa. To explain it at layman's term, since your insulin won't be spiking up sporadically throughout the day, your growth hormone will be going out gradually. When you mix it up with your working out routine, this will be a great way to increase your growth hormone.

There have been studies showing that intermittent fasting has increased growth hormone by up to four thousand percent, which is insane if you think about it. The growth hormone has many benefits, including more muscle mass, a higher rate of fat loss and the best of them all anti-aging effects. Meaning if these benefits sound useful to you, then you need to follow intermittent fasting and, moreover, make sure your insulin is in check.

## Muscle Mass and Intermittent Fasting Hunger

Many people who follow intermittent fasting, feel like they will lose muscle while following the eating protocol. However, the truth is they won't lose any muscle at all, and instead, they will gain a lot more muscle since their growth hormone will be going up.

Here's The thing, in order for you to lose muscle while intermittent fasting, you will have to fast for more than 3 days to see some loss. There have been studies showing that 48 Hours of fasting has had no effects on muscle loss. So if you're thinking about not following intermittent fasting because you might lose your muscle, then don't because you won't lose your muscle while following intermittent fasting. Instead, it's better for fat loss and will help you gain more muscle, and here's why. As we told you previously intermittent fasting has shown to increase growth hormone levels, growth hormone levels have also proved to increase muscle mass put two and two together you see a recipe to more muscle and less fat.

Now that we've discussed muscle mass and intermittent fasting, let's briefly touch upon hunger you might be experiencing while following intermittent fasting. For the first couple of weeks, he will notice some Hunger while fasting. It is incredibly reasonable to feel that way, just because your body is not used to intermittent fasting. Give it a couple of weeks, and you should be in a routine of intermittent fasting and not even feeling of hunger.

## Balancing Hunger While Fasting

Balancing hunger while fasting, is very easy to do later on in the stage. Although in the beginning, it would be tough for you to manage your hunger, there are some ways to avoid that, and we will show you how to do that. The first thing would be to start intermittent fasting slowly, and you need to make sure that intermittent fasting has been eased into because you don't want to give up midway while fasting. Perhaps starting with a skipping meal type of fasting or anything which seems natural to you is something you should start with. Another way to ensure that you don't notice any hunger while fasting is to make sure that you are drinking plenty of water.

There have been studies showing that when you drink more water suppresses your appetite, so make sure you're drinking much water during and after you're fast. The last one you can suppress hunger while fasting or balance it. I should say is to make sure that you drink more coffee and tea throughout the day. Not only will coffee and tea give you a lot more energy, but it would also help you to balance out your hunger. Coffee and tea have been shown to reduce hunger levels, merely have a couple of coffee throughout the day. Just make sure that there are no additives for the coffee, as we don't want to break her fast so I can see me something that has calories in them.

## Eating Enough to Break Your Fast

The truth is that you need to make sure that you are getting enough before you break your fast, the best way to do that is to count your calories. Counting calories isn't as hard as you think it is; the reason why it isn't so hard is there many tools you can use online to make sure that you're getting enough calories throughout the day. What intermittent fasting does merely allows you to eat at a particular time of the day. It tricks your body into thinking that they're in starvation mode when they're not.

Nonetheless, you can still get enough calories to put on muscle lose weight or to maintain. The way to do that is to break it into two big meals since you only have a particular time to get all your calories, but the main thing you need to make sure that you are eating enough before you break your fast. To make sure they are eating enough before you break your fast is to calculate all the meals that you are going to be having during your eating window. I figure out how many calories you need for your goals and then breaking into two meals. This will let you have enough food when you break your fast and not see any adverse effects that you might recognize from dieting. It is very common for people to undereating during intermittent fasting because they only have a specific time to eat food, make sure you're not making that mistake.

## Get Some Sleep

I'm sure you know the importance of getting enough sleep throughout the day, especially when intermittent fasting, you need to make sure they get enough sleep throughout the day. The reason why I need to get enough sleep is to ensure that your hormones are producing optimally throughout the day. When you're sleeping, not only recovering from the rest of the day but you're also boosting your growth hormone and other hormones that are related to health and wellness.

You need to make sure that you get enough sleep throughout the day, as we said before 6 to 8 hours is optimal for people looking to get the health benefits from sleeping. When intermittent fasting, in the beginning, you might find it hard to sleep. The reason why is because your adrenaline might be high throughout the day and will continue to stay that high later that night, a couple of ways to ensure they get enough sleep throughout the day while intermittent fasting is by perhaps meditating.

Meditation has shown to help people get into a calm mental state, which will help you sleep better. Please do whatever you have to do to get those 6 8 hours of sleep, as it is very crucial for your health and overall success following intermittent fasting.

## Autophagy

You might have heard claims such as intermittent fasting having anti-aging properties, and there is some truth behind it. When you are following an eating protocol related to fasting, your body will start a process known as autophagy. Autophagy is a process when your cells essentially eat themselves and produce newer and stronger ones. This process is known as autophagy. When you are eating regularly, your body has to work hard on digesting the foods which you are consuming and then doesn't have the time or energy to activate autophagy.

This is why you will see amazing results when intermittent fasting because when you are fasting, you are not digesting any food hence having more time for your body to activate the process of rejuvenating new cells. For you to see amazing results from autophagy, you will have to fast for at least 12 to 16 hours. The reason being is that your body will have burned out all the glycogen in your liver to get the process started, another thing to remember is to not fast for two days at a time, as this is when autophagy slowly drops. Overall if your goal is to live longer, you need to have an autophagy process running in a healthy manner, which fasting provides you.

## Other Tips

Now to close out this chapter, let's talk about a couple of things you need to consider when following intermittent fasting or some tips that might help you while observing intermittent fasting. The main thing that will help you when observing intermittent fasting is to make sure that everything is on point.

Make sure though your diet is okay, your sleep is in check and your exercising in check. When everything is in check, you will see the results that you are looking for. Another tip we would like to give you is to make sure that you ease into intermittent fasting. If you don't ease into it, chances are you might quit, and once you stopped, then there are lot fewer chances of you trying it again. Just start slowly, and increase your fast from there really feel of intermittent fasting before you start messing around with longer fasts. Before you start any of those, make sure you consult your physician or doctor to see if you're healthy enough to follow intermittent fasting.

# Chapter 6: How to Make Intermittent Fasting a Lifestyle

By now, you should know many things that are related to intermittent fasting, so let's talk about the steps you need to take before you start your intermittent fasting diet.

## Before You Get Started

Before you get started, there are a couple of things to understand about intermittent fasting. The first thing is going to be making sure that intermittent fasting is followed the right way, as described in this book. If you don't do it right, then chances of you achieving your goals will go down significantly, so make sure you read this book very carefully before you start any fat intermittent fasting diet protocol.

## Consult a Health Physician

Before you start any diet, you need to consult with your position. As we talked about before how intermittent fasting cannot be suited for some people out there, oh, so it is in your best interest to figure out if you are well enough to follow intermittent fasting. Ideally, you want to consult with someone whom you can trust, perhaps your doctor or a dietitian. However, whatever you do, you make sure that you consult with a professional who knows what they're doing since we don't see what you look like or what your health complications are we can tell you if you're fit enough for intermittent fasting or not. If you aren't fit enough for intermittent fasting, then perhaps try something new.

## Keep It Easy

Keeping it easy one of the best things you can do to your body Because the truth is it needs to feel less like a chore and more like a lifestyle, so if you want to be successful in this, then it needs to feel comfortable. If you feel like intermittent fasting is a chore for you from the get-go, then the chances of you continuing with intermittent fasting will go down drastically. Whatever you do, make sure the intermittent fasting feels comfortable for you and that it is not a chore but more so of a lifestyle.

Now there's a couple of ways to keep it easy, and the first way would be to start slow. We have to explain to you how to start easy, so start with that and then move on to the big stuff. Overall you want to make intermittent fasting and easy manageable part of your life, and you have to figure out how you're going to do that. We can give you some pointers and some tricks on how to do that, but it is for you to find out what works for you and what doesn't.

## Keep It Simple

Please don't make things harder than they're supposed to be, especially when you're intermittent fasting. It is straightforward to make things hard when following intermittent fasting, as there many things to consider and many things to do. The best thing you can do is keep things simple; the way to keep things simple is by not overthinking stuff. By that, I mean, not overthinking how much food you're missing while fasting or what kind of foods you will be eating when you break your fast. Just take it one step at a time, when you start taking one step at a time is a lot easier for you to continue with intermittent fasting and it won't feel like such a chore.

Also, when you try to keep things simple, you need to realize that it is in your best interest to stay away from external information which might throw you off. Such as new diet fads that are coming out, make sure you stay in your lane and follow intermittent fasting for the time being. Please stick to the plan, do not deviate from it, and finally, keep things simple.

## What Time Will You Begin?

Now we come on to the main question, the main question being when will you start intermittent fasting and the simple answer to that is whatever time feels right to you. Here's the thing, whatever time fits your schedule and all your needs will work the best, the truth is that intermittent fasting doesn't have a specific time when you fast and when you don't fast. If you're following a 16 hour fast, then you can quickly start your fast at 8 p.m. and break it at 12 p.m. the next day, or whatever time works for you.

Just make sure that you're fast ends closer to your work out time. Especially for someone looking to put on muscle, make sure whenever you work out, you are breaking your fast right after it. This will ensure that you get enough protein in your system to build a muscle back, which you broke down, this isn't necessary, but it is an ideal situation. Figure out when you work out, and map out the times he will be fasting and the times you will be eating, and you have your fasting protocol.

## Choose Which Days to Fast

Depending on the type of intermittent fasting you're going to be falling, we need to pick out what days you will be fasting what Daisy will not be fasting. Ideally, you want to pick a day when you're doing a lot less work to fast, and when you have more stuff at hand, you can decide to not fast on that day.

Just make sure whatever day you pick, that it is comfortable for you to fast, then it is on other days. Like I said before, there are no restrictions on the time or the date when you're fasting or non-fasting. As long as you get the things done, you're fasting endeavors would be a good and overall help you achieve your goal.

## Forgive Your Slip-Ups

There will be many times that you will be slipping up, but don't worry that happens to everyone. Here's the thing following a routine and sticking to it as a good thing, but we are humans, and we will slip up time and time again, it makes you feel any better I have as well. So when you're fasting, don't think of you slip up those failures feel of it as a stepping stone. Maybe your body needs a break, which is why you had that stuff up.

Moreover, once you do have your slip-ups forgive yourself and move on and start over again. Eventually, you will get to the point that it becomes more for lifestyle, and you won't have any slip-ups anymore. Just keep going at it, don't give up, and you will be fine.

## What Is Your Purpose

Many people when they're starting intermittent fasting, and they figure out the meaning. The truth is that you need to find out why you're following intermittent fasting and what your goals are. So if your goal is to lose weight, they need to make sure that that is your only call, and then once you figure out what your goal is, you need to pick a plan which works the best for you.

In the later chapters we will show you how to pick a plan out for your goals, just realize that you will still notice many health benefits from all the intermittent fasting, but you got to recognize on some intermittent fasting Protocols are better suited for people who are looking to lose weight rather than see some health benefits.

## What Are Your Concerns

You have to forget all your worries when following intermittent fasting, and going to it stress-free. If you have any questions or concerns regarding intermittent fasting, find out what they are and figure them out at how you are going to fix it. Most of the things regarding intermittent fasting will be covered in this book. However, you need to do your research and find out what works for you and what doesn't.

## Take Precautions

As we mentioned to you before, you need to take precautions when you're falling intermittent fasting. You need to realize when you're not feeling well when intermittent fasting, which means you need to understand your body.

If you ever feel like you, in spite of fasting is causing you more harm and fewer benefits than in his stop intermittent fasting done in there. If you consult with the doctor, then you will know precisely if intermittent fasting is the answer for you or not. Just make sure whatever you were doing, is healthy for you. Taking precautions include many things, but more specifically, you are prepared for what is coming when intermittent fasting.

## Pregnancy

If you're pregnant, then you should not follow intermittent fasting. The reason why I should not have intermittent fasting, it's because your body needs regular food all the time to feed you and your infant, so if you are pregnant, then you should not follow intermittent fasting as it is not only in healthy for you, but it will be unhealthy for a child as well.

The chances of you giving up when intermittent fasting while pregnant will be extremely high, the simple reason why is because it isn't safe for pregnant women.

## Diabetes

One of the great benefits of intermittent fasting is that it reduces the risk of many diseases, more specifically reduces the risk of diabetes. However, if you already have diabetes, then you should not be falling intermittent fasting; here's why.

When you diabetic, you're taking something called insulin; when you are taking insulin, you need regular food throughout the day are you all go until glycemic coma, And once you going to glycemic coma, chances of surviving would be slim to none.

Believe it or not, when intermittent fasting when you're on a diabetic prescription, it could be very deadly. So if you have diabetes are facing any health issues for the small consult with the doctor, and sing of all make sure your novel intermittent fasting as it can be deadly

## Electrolyte Imbalance

When you're falling intermittent fasting, the chances of you noticing electrolyte imbalances will be very high. You need to make sure they getting enough electrolytes throughout the day to make sure that your body is functioning correctly. Sometimes people drink electrolyte drinks while following intermittent fasting, which we don't recommend since I can break your fast.

However, when you do break your fast to get how some electrolyte drinks to replenish electrolytes. Some of the ways to tell the electrolytes are low is to see how you feel throughout the day if you were noticing joint pains lower energy than trans are electrolytes are a little bit on the lower side to make sure that you get that checked. Overall, make sure that once you do break your fast to get all the electrolytes that you need.

## Start Intermittent Fasting Quickly

Many beginners make the mistake of starting intermittent fasting way too fast, and when they begin to quickly, it becomes unsustainable for them to continue with intermittent fasting. If you have begun anything immediately, you might have noticed that it became tough for you to follow, which led to you not continuing. The same goes for intermittent fasting, and you need to make sure you take the right steps before you jump into following intermittent fasting. With that being said, let's talk about many ways beginner intermittent fasters tend to start too quickly. The first mistake they make is by picking a fasting protocol which is way out of their Realm.

As we talked about before, you need to ease into intermittent fasting, especially if you're women. You cannot expect to fast for 24 hours when you have never even fasted in your life, so start small. It is always recommended that women begin with 12-hour fast, or if that sounds too intense for you can begin to by meal skipping. You simply have to make sure that, whatever you follow, it is done in a gradual manner, so you don't quit. Another way people tend to start intermittent fasting too quickly is by not Consulting the doctor.

Believe it or not, their chances that you might not be healthy enough to follow intermittent fasting.

That is why it is recommended that you consult a doctor before starting to fast. For example, if you are 2 diabetics, you are not advised to start intermittent fasting. There are many health complications which not allow you to follow intermittent fasting; that is why we always recommend you ask a doctor before you start intermittent fasting, or it can be very devastating.

Beginners also tend to extend the fasting window very quickly; if you haven't fasted for more than 4 weeks comfortably, then it is not recommended to extend the fasting window. We need to take into consideration that for beginners, going from 12 hours to 16 hours can be a drastic difference. That is why it is always recommended that you stick with a fasting protocol for an extended period of time ideally for four weeks. If you make the jump of increasing hours too soon, you will notice it becomes very hard for you to continue on with fasting, and you might give up.

## Ignore What for When

One mistake that many people following intermittent fasting make is to ignore what for when. For you to be successful with intermittent fasting, you need to make sure you don't overlook what for when. What do I mean by what for when is simple, ignoring what to do and what not to do when intermittent fasting. We will talk about things to avoid and the things not to avoid when intermittent fasting. More specifically, we will teach you how to listen to your body.

Ignoring what for when is merely a metaphor, nonetheless an important one. First of all, when intermittent fasting doesn't jump too quickly from fasts to fasts. Most beginners make the mistake of not riding out the protocol for a substantial amount of time before they jump to conclusions. Make sure that you have done at least four weeks of following this protocol as it will show you how your body reacts to this fasting method. The next thing to make sure of would be to understand how your body reacts to certain types of fasting, as it is very important that you know so.

Before you jump the guns of upping the fasting difficulty, make sure you know how your body works. You need to remember that your body is more important than your goals, so whatever you do, you need to be aware of what your body is telling you. Don't do anything which makes you feel like you are harming your body, and as always, consult with your physician before you start a fast.

# Chapter 7: Intermittent Fasting and Fitness

When following intermittent fasting, you have to keep in mind that even though you are eating very healthy and that you are taking care of your body, having a good workout routine is recommended. Once you figured out what kind of intermittent fasting plan you're going to be following, make sure that you get a workout plan that will help you to put on muscle or lose body fat whichever your goal is.

One of the great amazing things about intermittent fasting is that you can lose weight or gain muscle while following this method, which is why many people consider intermittent fasting one of the best eating plans to follow, for overall health and wellness. By now, you know everything about intermittent fasting and how you should be following, especially for women, as it is different from men when it comes to intermittent fasting. To understand how to stay healthy when intermittent fasting, there are some things you need to take care of before you start intermittent fasting. The first one would be to make sure that you have a proper workout plan based on your goals, there are many workout plans which you can find online that will help you to come up with a workout plan based on your goals. Keep in mind that you will have to work hard to come up with a workout plan if you're not an expert. If you can afford to get a personal trainer, then get one, as it will help you create a great workout plan for your needs. However, finding a workout plan online isn't so hard, and you can do so by looking up online for a bit.

Another aspect you need to make sure when intermittent fasting is that you need to take care of your diet, even though you are allowed to eat whatever you want when intermittent fasting you need to make sure that your diet is a lot healthier if your goal is to lose weight. Don't get me wrong, and you will still lose weight when following intermittent fasting; however, making sure that you are eating very healthy, then you will see better results overall. Finally, you need to make sure that you're taking care of yourself internally. Make sure they are getting enough micronutrients throughout the day to support your health.

Another thing to keep in mind would be that you will lose fat most of the time when fasting instead of the weight. Keep in mind, and When fasting, you will gain muscle and lose fat, which might not make you lose weight but instead fat. As always, do body measurements instead of bodyweight check overall.

There are many ways to go about it, but one of the best ways to go about it would be to take multivitamins during you're eating window. Keep in mind that if you take multivitamins when you are fasting will break the fast, so make sure that you're not taking multivitamins during your fast but in fact, after your fast. Finally, make sure that you do everything in conjunction if your goal is to see amazing results. There is no better way to see results, and if you combine all three aspects, then you will be in a much better place to truly reap the benefits out of it

When following intermittent fasting, one of the main things you need to consider would be diet exercise and rest. In this chapter, we will go into depts on how you can ensure that all of the things listed above are in check. Many of you might be falling back on either three of these aspects; the sooner you realize which one it is and fix it the better.

## Diet and Nutrition

In the previous chapter, we already talked about the importance of diet and nutrition; let's further discuss it to ensure that you are optimizing this aspect as well. Having the right diet and nutrition can either break you or make you in the realm of fitness and health. The simplest way to ensure that your diet and nutrition is on point is to keep it simple, by that I mean not following any crazy diets which will hinder your goals and success.

The best way to go about it would be just to eat healthy foods during your eating window. Please do not make your food intake very complicated; if your goal is to lose weight, merely being a little bit of caloric deficit and eat good vegetables and meat will do the trick. This will provide you with optimal nutrition while striving for you towards your goals. The reason why we keep bringing up diet and nutrition, Is to show you that you can follow intermittent fasting without overthinking. If your diet or nutrition plan is too complicated for you and becomes a chore, then chances are you're not following the right strategy. The next time you're planning out your food intake, make sure that this isn't a chore for you and More so of a lifestyle.

## How Intermittent Fasting Affects Your Body

Intermittent fasting works in a unique way, so let's talk about it. When you're following an intermittent fasting type of eating protocol, you are going to a starvation mode. When you're into starvation mode, your body thinks that it's not getting enough food, and therefore it starts breaking down your fat stores.

The same thing would happen to our ancestors. They would go without food for a couple of days, and once they did find food they would eat much food to store it into body fat stores so they can use it later on. We are merely following a diet, which was used by our ancestors. Believe it or not, there are a lot healthier than us, and they didn't have any diseases such as diabetes and so on.

Nonetheless, let's get into the science of intermittent fasting. When you are fasting, your body will burn off all the glycogen and your bloodstreams for a couple of hours. Once it has burnt out all the glycogen in your bloodstream, it will start to use your fat stores for energy. Which is where the magic happens, you will burn more fat throughout the day than you would following any other diet, which makes intermittent fasting, one of the best diets to follow if your goal is to lose fat or to lower the risk of diseases.

## Eating Wrong Foods Can Counter Those Effects

Eating the wrong foods can counter those effects during intermittent fasting. Even though when you're following intermittent fasting, you're allowed to eat whatever you want. However, that doesn't mean it is the most optimal way to go about it, here's the thing if you want to ensure that you're not countering the effects from intermittent fasting then you need to eat the right foods.

Since you already know the right foods to eat when intermittent fasting, let's talk about the wrong foods that you shouldn't eat when you're following an intermittent fasting type of protocol. The first thing you should not eat would be anything that would be considered junk food, even though most people have seen success through eating junk food while intermittent fasting. We don't recommend that you do the same, because the chances are you will store that food into fats quickly, then you would eating healthy foods. Another reason why you should not eat junk food while intermittent fasting is because it would not help you lower the risk of any diseases. Even though intermittent fasting is a powerful way to reduce the risk of diseases, it can't be countered without the consumption of healthy foods.

On the other hand, eating junk food by itself will increase the risk of heart diseases and diabetes. To keep everything simple, stay away from food, which would be considered fast foods. Once you manage to do that, you will be in a lot better place.

## Important Food Groups for Nutrition

There are many essential food groups to consider when following intermittent fasting. To keep things very simple, eat foods that were available thousands of years ago. These include meats, vegetables, and some grains here and there. The thing that you need to consider to eat foods which are low on the glycemic index, so you don't increase your insulin levels when you do eat those foods.

When you spike your insulin level consistently, you put yourself at risk of attracting type 2 diabetes. This is why you need to research the types of food you're eating, so make sure whatever you're eating has a low glycemic index. Most of the time, foods such as brown rice, meat, and vegetables tend to have a very low glycemic index.

Meaning they will not spike your insulin very quickly, and it will take time for you to burn off those calories from the food giving you a sustained amount of energy throughout the day. This is where you want to be when following intermittent fasting, and you need to have a sustained amount of energy throughout the day.

The main three food groups of nutrition would be carbohydrates protein and fats. It would be best if you made sure that all three of these are coming from good healthy food. It would help if you were careful more on the carbohydrates side of the nutrition, as are many carbohydrates that will spike your insulin very quickly. Simply eat carbohydrates, which are low on the glycemic index, and you will be fine.

## Does Intermittent Fasting and Exercise Go Together

Many people feel that intermittent fasting exercise does not go together, just because of the fact that you're starving yourself throughout the day. However, the truth is when following an intermittent fasting type of protocol, you have terrific workouts, and there's a reason behind it.

When you're intermittent fasting, your body goes into starvation mode, when your body is in the starvation mode it raises your adrenaline which is why some people notice better mental focus while fasting. When your adrenaline goes up, you will have more energy to do physical tasks because your body feels like it needs to be fighting for food, which is why you will have a lot of energy throughout the day, especially when you going to work out. From personal experience, I can tell you that I've had one of my best workouts while following intermittent fasting and that too while I was in the fast. The best part about working out while intermittent fasting is that you will burn fat for energy instead of glycogen for energy.

Meaning that you will actually gain more fat loss benefits from working out while intermittent fasting. Some have said that intermittent fasting lowers their strength levels, but it is not noticeable if you're not a powerlifter. If your goal is merely to lose weight that intermittent fasting is a great idea to be falling while working out.

## Go for High-Intensity Workouts After Eating

Here is the truth, the best way to burn fat when falling intermittent fasting is to follow a high-intensity type of workout plan. When you follow a high-intensity kind of workout plan, you'll actually burn a lot more calories for an extended period. Ideally, should be working out right after you have broken your fast, this will put you in a position where you have some food in you to burn off. High-intensity workouts work great if your goal is to have better cardiovascular health and to burn off some fat.

Ideally should be doing a cardio workout, at least three to four times a week, to ensure that your fat is actually melting off, but in conjunction with that, you need to make sure that your workouts are high intensity. This will not only burn off more fat, but it will raise your hormones, which will help you live a better life or healthier life, I should say. The next time you're planning out your workouts, make sure that they are high intensity and short. This will ensure that you are getting closer to your goals every day without leaving any stones unturned.

## Eat High Protein Meals

You might have noticed that many people in the fitness industry suggests that others eat high protein meals. There's a reason for that, and the reason is that protein is one of the best macro-nutrients if you're looking to burn fat and to live a healthier life. Let's get into the Science as to why protein is essential when following an intermittent fasting type of protocol, the first thing that protein does is preserve your muscle.

When you have more muscle mass new body, you will burn more fat. Therefore it is essential to have more protein to prevent muscle loss. Another thing protein is really good at is burning off fat, protein is the macronutrient that requires the most calories to digest. Which is why we need more protein to burn fat because it takes so much energy to digest the calories and fats.

Another great thing that protein does is that it will not raise your insulin levels, Unlike carbohydrates protein does not increase your insulin levels when you eat it. which is why it is a great idea to have more protein in your diet because you will get the energy and it will not raise your insulin levels. If your goal is to lose weight, look a lot better, and live a healthy life. Then you need to have enough protein in your diet. Protein is the building block to your body, and it will build muscle; it will burn fat and, most importantly, keep you healthy for the days to come. Make sure that you are getting enough protein in your diet.

## Rest

We talked about diet and working out so far, and the truth is those are one of the most important things to consider when following intermittent fasting or any diet for that matter. However, the most critical thing we tend to overlook is the rest. If you're not resting enough, then you will not see results are you looking for.

There needs to be a right balance between exercising and rest, which is what we will talk about in the section of the book. Ideally, you should be resting at least twice a week from your workouts, so you should work out no more than five times a week throughout the day, and that includes your cardio and weight training workouts. When you don't rest, your body will counter-react to the stimulus you are providing it with to put on muscle and lose fat. If you don't want that to happen, make sure you give yourself twice a week of rest. Another form of rest would be sleep.

You need to ensure that you are getting an ample amount of sleep throughout the days, this will also help you recover from your workouts, more importantly, it will help you produce the optimal amount of hormones that you need for healthy body function. Some people say that you need 8 to 10 hours of sleep, but the truth is you can survive with 6 to 8 hours of sleep. Just make sure that you're getting enough sleep to recover your body from working out and the daily stress that you might have acquired. Overall, rest is an essential part of your fitness and health goals, so the last thing you need to do is overlook it.

# Chapter 8: Common Mistakes to Avoid

Many people who are just starting their fasting cycle, tend to make beginner's mistakes, which can result in goals not being achieved and many other hosts of things. In this chapter, we will talk about the main mistakes most beginners make when they first start fasting. If you are just starting off with intermittent fasting, chances are you will make those mistakes. Meaning, in order for it to not happen, it is best that we talk about it and show you ways to combat it. With that being said, let's talk about the first mistake.

## Eat Too Much During the Eating Window or Too Little

People make the mistake of eating too much or too little when following intermittent fasting, and the truth is it is straightforward to do either. People who are looking to lose weight will eat less during their eating window, thinking that it will help you lose more body fat. Whereas overeating will not make up for all the fasting, you did throughout the day. This is why it is imperative that you do none, so in this section, we will teach you how to make sure you aren't doing either when following an intermittent fasting protocol.

The first way to not mess up on eating too much would be to make sure that you are counting your macros. This is one of the best ways to make sure you stay on track with your eating habits during your fasting windows. When you have calculated your macros and following them accordingly, you will have a lot better chance of not under-eating or overeating during your eating window. Another way to make sure that you are not overeating is to eat slowly, and many people tend to get extremely excited when they see food in front of them during their eating window. It is best advised that you don't indulge in them and more than you should.

That is why it is essential that you control your cravings; we have taught you how to do that in the previous chapters. Now, even though fasting allows you to eat whatever you want when you break your fast it still important to make sure you eat correctly. You see, if you try and eat junk food and try and hit your macros, it would be tough for you not to overeat. Let me explain how that works, as there is something called a high glycemic carb, which most of the junk foods. What these high glycemic carbs are responsible for is digesting very quickly in your body, which spikes the insulin very fast.

When you absorb and shuttle the foods to quickly as you would with junk food, you will get hungry very fast, which would make you overeat. This is why it is best advised that you eat foods that have a lower glycemic index like most healthy meals tend to have. Another thing these healthy foods will help you with would be the fiber, making you feel fuller throughout the day. Now that we know how to not overeat let's talk about how to make sure that you aren't under-eating. The first way to make sure that you aren't under-eating would be by counting macros; this will help you make sure that you are hitting all your calories for the day. Counting macros will ensure you don't under-eat, and you don't overeat, it goes hand in hand.

Now, this is the only way to avoid under-eating. Let's talk about some of the signs you might be experiencing if you under-eat when fasting. The first sign you might notice is that you feel very weak when working out if you follow a workout plan you will notice that your strength has gone down which is a tail-tail sign that you are under-eating. Another way to tell that you are under-eating is if you notice that you feel less energy throughout the day, rather than feeling more energy. One of the many benefits of intermittent fasting is the fact that you can get a lot more energy, but it won't work if you are under-eating. So by now, you can tell that overeating and under-eating isn't optimal for fasting. Which is why you need to make sure that you stay on track with your macros when fasting, the other tips we gave you work great as well.

But do whatever works for you in order to ensure that you aren't under-eating or overeating, and there are millions of ways to go about it. Find an eating routine which helps you feel full, and allows you to eat just the right amount of calories to where you are getting closer to your goals instead of drifting away from them if your goal is weight loss or muscle gains you need to make sure your calories are the right amount. Don't make this beginner's mistake as you will regret it, and now you have the tools to ensure you don't make these mistakes.

## Not Drinking Enough Water

Drinking water is crucial when you are intermittent fasting, is there a lot of benefits to drinking water. It also helps you care about your appetite. We will talk about the reasons why you should be drinking more water when intermittent fasting, and also show you why you might not be drinking enough water and techniques to allow you to drink more water when fasting. Many people know that water is very beneficial to humans, water help to detox your body clean out your system and also helps you curb appetite. It is crucial that you're drinking more water when fasting. Believe it or not, most of the time, you're drinking a lot less water than you required to be drinking. One of the best rules of thumb to follow when you are drinking water, so drink 1 oz per pound of bodyweight, so if you weigh 150 lb. you should be drinking 150 ounces of water. Especially when you're intermittent fasting, as water will help you forget about food.

Many people know that when you're fasting, especially in the beginning, you tend to crave a lot of food. What water will do is help you curb that appetite, so you don't break you're fast prematurely, another thing water will do detoxify your body. When your fasting, you're already detoxing a lot of things; if you add more water to it will help you detox your body even further, making it a lot more healthy environment for you. Water will also increase your brainpower and productivity. As you know, intermittent fasting has shown to improve mental focus so once you add more water to your daily routine, you will notice more focused throughout the day.

Another thing water helps you with is that it helps you lose bodyweight. If you started intermittent fasting in the hopes of losing weight, then you need to drink more water. What water does is increase your metabolism, which equals more calories burnt throughout the day. Water will also help you clean out your complexion, so if that's what you're looking for then water will help you with that. Intermittent fasting has shown to improve with your digestive system, but once you add a sufficient amount of water to it will boost it further. Many people know that regularity in the very important thing when it comes to a healthy body, why do I help you with regularity which will equal a better digestive system and overall well-being. Water will also help you boost your immune system, as it enables you to clean out your toxins.

When incorporated with intermittent fasting, drink more water to boost your immune system. When fasting, you might notice headaches, especially in the beginning. If you drink a sufficient amount of water throughout the day, you will not notice headaches. Headaches are one of the biggest concerns when fasting; many people notice headaches and to avoid that, you should start drinking more water. Another matter that you might notice when fasting is cramping, more specifically, muscle cramps. One of the ways to prevent it is to drink more water. Now I can keep going on with the benefits of drinking more water, but you get the idea to drink more water in order to avoid side effects from fasting that you might see.

One of the ways to ensure that you drink more water is to buy a water bottle with markings on it. First, figure out how much water you need throughout the day and make sure you achieve your goal of drinking a set amount of water. Another way to ensure that you drink more water is to set alarms. What many people do, set alarms on this Smartphone, and when the alarm goes off, they drink a glass of water. You can do the same thing to ensure they drink enough water throughout the day, just calculate the number of glasses you need to achieve your water intake goal and then set your timer.

Choose whichever method you want to make sure that you're drinking enough water throughout the day. Not drinking enough water is one of the biggest mistakes most people make. Our body is made up of around 70% water, and to ignore that and not drink enough water and hinder your progress. Make sure you're drinking enough water, during your fast and after you break your fast. To ensure that you are optimizing your fasting endeavors and getting closer to your goals.

We have now officially completed the book, hope you learned a lot from it as it was our goal to ensure that no stones where unturned. This final chapter has to be one of the most important ones, as it helps you figure out any mistakes you might make in the beginning. Many books don't cover mistakes that beginners might make when following intermittent fasting, and that is why we had to write a chapter especially on it.

We understand that fasting can be confusing and hard at first, so it is essential that you are aware of the mistakes you might or might not make. Please make sure that you have understood all the things you should so and the things you shouldn't be doing. Just be aware of the fact that there might be many things which might go wrong in the beginning, simply learn from your mistakes, and keep moving on forward.

Don't let small mistakes stop you from achieving your dream body, and helping you live a healthier life overall. If you need extra motivation, ask a friend to keep you on track, always let them know how important it is for you to not give up on this journey. But once again, listen to your body if you feel like fasting is harming your body then stop. As your body is more important than anything else, which is why we recommend getting blood work done by a professional always before you start any plan.

# Conclusion

Thank you so much for reading the book. *Intermittent Fasting Guide for Weight Loss: The Ultimate Beginners Guide for Weight Loss, Heal Your Body, and Live a Healthy Lifestyle while Eating Your Favorite Foods (Includes 5:2 and 16:8 Method).* As you can see, we went through a lot when it comes to intermittent fasting, and we taught you how not only to start intermittent fasting but how to avoid any risk arising along with it. Understanding how occasional works is significant, and you should have a clear idea of how it works.

Moreover, we also taught you how to pick the right plan for your lifestyle. Choosing the right plan for your lifestyle is very important when it comes to intermittent fasting, which is why we made it so easy for you when it comes to picking out the right plan. More specifically, we also gave you a workout plan and an idea on how to work out when it comes to intermittent fasting and healthy living. Overall, this book should give you a clear idea of how to follow intermittent fasting without wasting any time or effort. If you enjoyed this book, then make sure that you recommended it to your friends and family as it could help us much.

www.ingramcontent.com/pod-product-compliance
Lightning Source LLC
Chambersburg PA
CBHW070352220526
45467CB00001B/351